Notice:

e the information contained within this
s for educational and entertainment purposes
fort has been executed to present accurate,
, and reliable, complete information. No
s of any kind are declared or implied. Readers
dge that the author is not engaging in the
g of legal, financial, medical, or professional
he content within this book has been derived
arious sources. Please consult a licensed
onal before attempting any techniques outlined
book.
ding this document, the reader agrees that under
umstances is the author responsible for any losses,
or indirect, which are incurred as a result of the
f the information contained within this document,
ding, but not limited to, — errors, omissions, or
uracies.

Vege

50 Quick a.

America

Table of contents

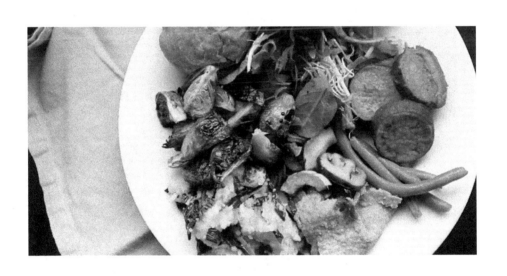

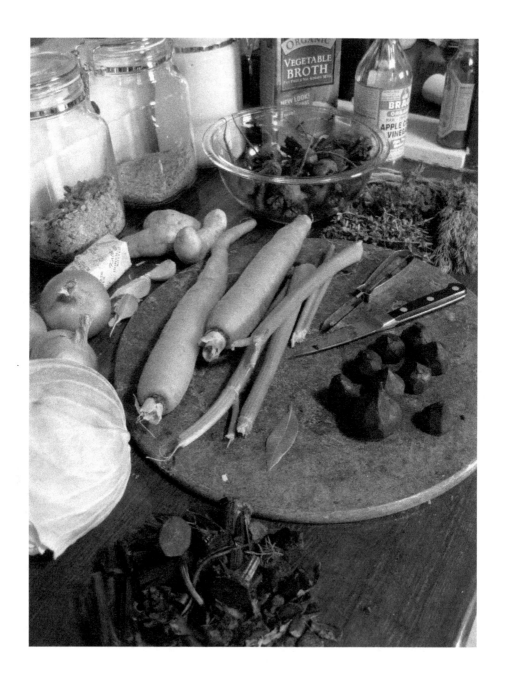

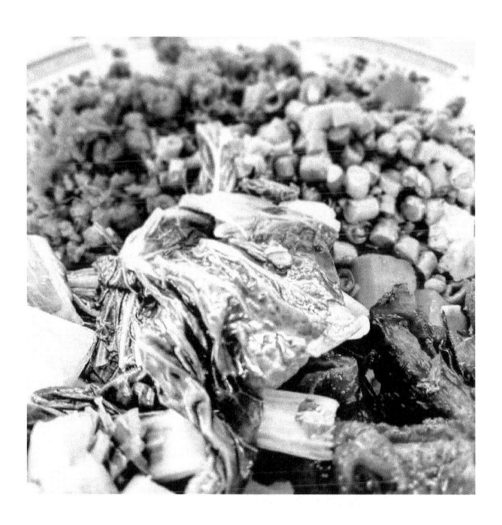

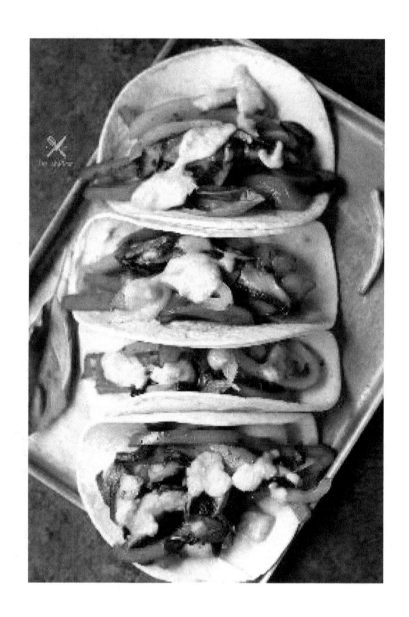

1.Scallions Broccoli

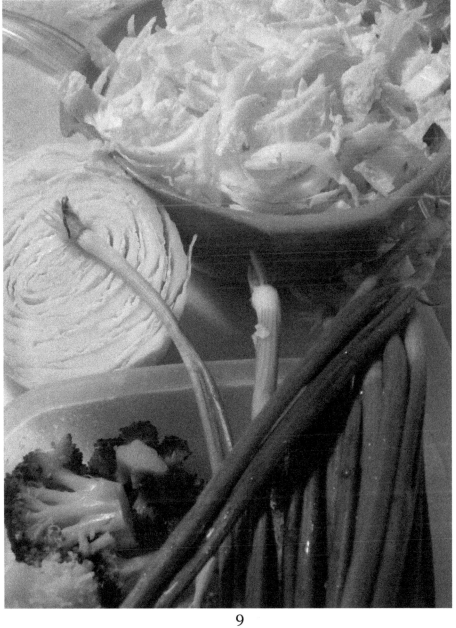

Prep Time:5 m | **Cook Time:** 15 m | **Servings:** 4

- 1-pound broccoli, roughly chopped
- 1 tablespoon olive oil
- 1 teaspoon salt
- 2 oz scallions, chopped

1. Mix broccoli with olive oil and salt.
2. Put it in the air fryer basket and cook it for 5 minutes per side at 365F.
3. Then sprinkle the broccoli with scallions and cook the meal for 5 minutes more.

Per Serving: calories 73, fat 3.9, fiber 3.3, carbs 8.6, protein 3.4

2.Cheddar Rutabaga

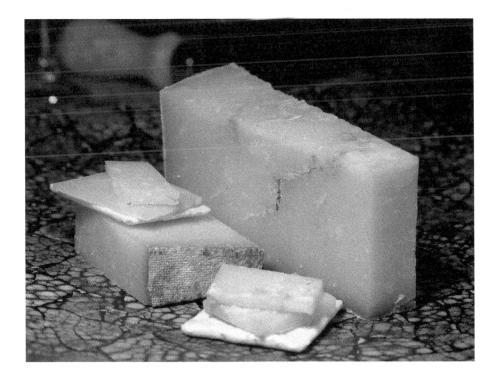

Prep Time: 12 m | **Cook Time:** 8 m | **Servings:** 2

- 6 oz rutabaga, chopped
- 2 oz Cheddar cheese, grated
- 1 tablespoon coconut oil
- ½ teaspoon dried cilantro
- ½ teaspoon salt
- ½ teaspoon onion powder
- 3 tablespoons coconut cream

1. Mix rutabaga with coconut oil, dried cilantro, salt, and onion powder.
2. Then add coconut cream and put the vegetables in the air fryer.
3. Cook them at 360F for 4 minutes per side.
4. Top the cooked rutabaga with Cheddar cheese.

Per Serving: calories 257, fat 21.7, fiber 2.7, carbs 9, protein 8.7

3.Chili Cauliflower

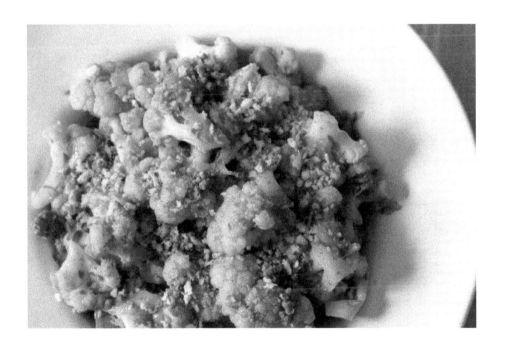

Prep Time:5 m | **Cook Time:** 15 m | **Servings:** 4

- 1-pound cauliflower florets
- 2 tablespoons sesame oil
- 2 tablespoons keto hot sauce
- 3 tablespoons lemon juice
- ½ teaspoon white pepper

1. Mix sesame oil with lemon juice, hot sauce, and white pepper.
2. Then mix cauliflower florets with the lemon juice mixture and put in the air fryer.
3. Cook them at 360F for 7 minutes per side.
4. Then cook the cauliflower for 1 minute at 400F.

Per Serving: calories 92, fat 7, fiber 3, carbs 6.4, protein 2.4

4.Coated Jicama

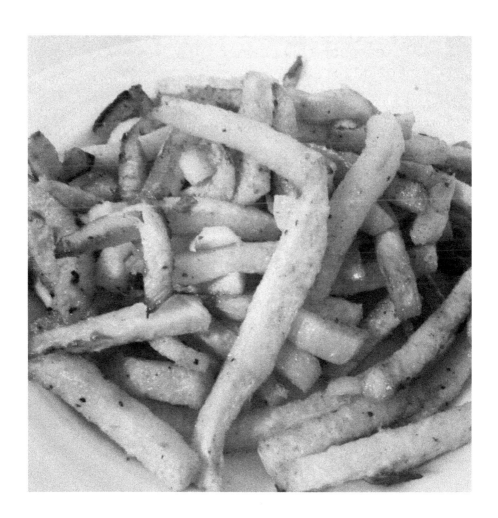

Prep Time:15 m | **Cook Time:** 7 | **Servings:** 5

- 15 oz jicama, peeled, cut into sticks
- 1 egg, beaten
- ¼ cup heavy cream
- ½ cup coconut shred
- 1 teaspoon chili powder
- Cooking spray

1. Mix egg with heavy cream and chili powder.
2. Dip the jicama sticks in the egg mixture and coat them in the coconut shred.
3. Put the coated jicama in the air fryer and spray with cooking spray.
4. Cook the meal at 390F for 7 minutes.

Per Serving: calories 121, fat 8.6, fiber 5.4, carbs 10.2, protein 2.4

5.Jarlsberg Cauliflower and Broccoli

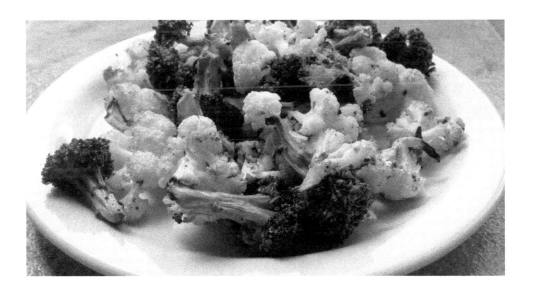

Prep Time:5 m | **Cook Time:** 15 m | **Servings:** 4

- 10 oz broccoli, chopped
- 10 oz cauliflower, chopped
- 4 oz Jarlsberg cheese, grated
- 2 tablespoons apple cider vinegar
- 1 tablespoon avocado oil

1. Mix broccoli with cauliflower, apple cider vinegar, and avocado oil.
2. Put the vegetables in the air fryer and top with Jarlsberg cheese.
3. Cook the meal at 365F for 15 minutes.

Per Serving: calories 149, fat 8.8, fiber 3.8, carbs 8.7, protein 10.5

6.Zucchini Noodles

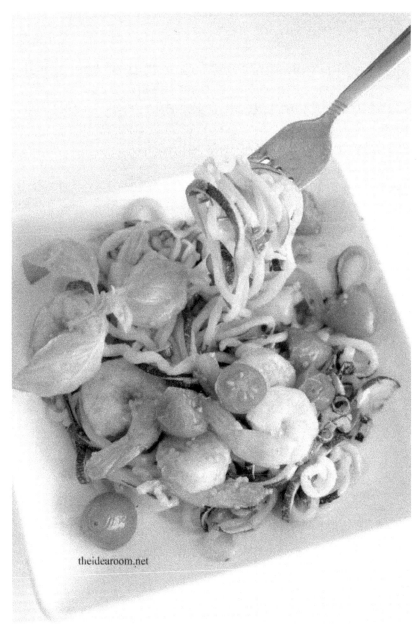

theidearoom.net

Prep Time:19 m | **Cook Time:** 5 m | **Servings:** 4

- 3 zucchinis, trimmed
- 1 tablespoon coconut oil
- 1 oz Parmesan, grated

1. Spiralize the zucchinis with the help of the spiralizer and mix with coconut oil and parmesan.
2. Put the mixture in the air fryer and cook at 360F for 5 minutes.
3. Carefully mix the cooked noodles.

Per Serving: calories 76, fat 5.2, fiber 1.6, carbs 5.2, protein 4.1

7.Broccoli Steaks

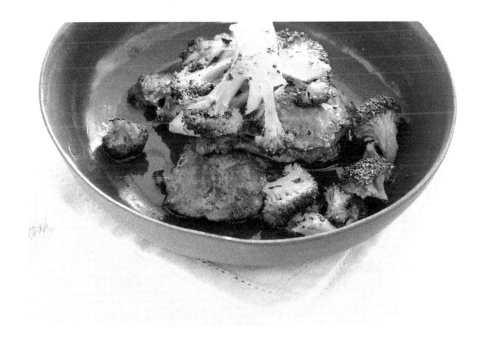

Prep Time:5 m | **Cook Time:** 12 m | **Servings:** 4

- 2-pound broccoli head
- 1 tablespoon coconut oil, melted
- 1 teaspoon garlic powder
- ½ teaspoon dried oregano

1. Slice the broccoli head into steaks.
2. Then rub them with coconut oil, garlic powder, and dried oregano.
3. Put the broccoli steaks in the air fryer and cook them at 365F for 6 minutes per side.

Per Serving: calories 40, fat 3.5, fiber 0.7, carbs 2.1, protein 0.7

8.Eggplant Slices

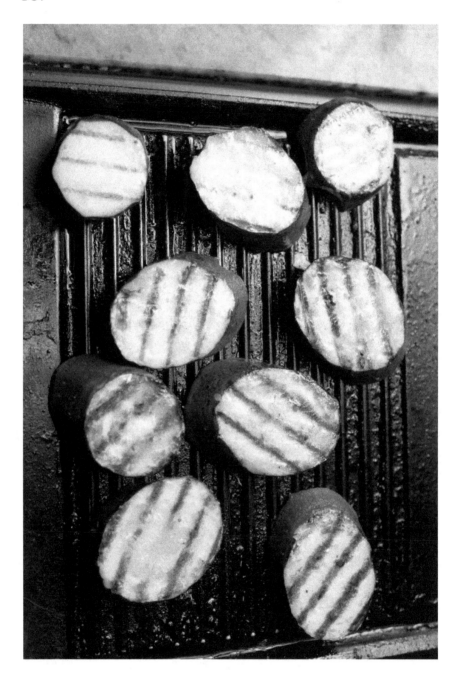

Prep Time:14 m | **Cook Time:** 14 m | **Servings:** 2

- 1 large eggplant, trimmed, peeled
- 1 teaspoon salt
- 1 teaspoon minced garlic
- Cooking spray

1. Slice the eggplant and sprinkle with minced garlic, salt, and cooking spray.
2. Then, put the eggplant slices in the air fryer and cook them for 7 minutes per side at 350F.

Per Serving: calories 59, fat 0.4, fiber 8.1, carbs 13.9, protein 2.3

9.Cauliflower Steaks

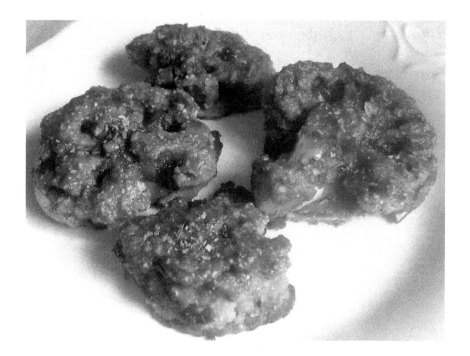

Prep Time:10 m | **Cook Time:** 14 m | **Servings:** 4

- 1.5-pound cauliflower head
- 1 tablespoon sesame oil
- 1 teaspoon ground turmeric
- 1 teaspoon dried dill

1. Cut the cauliflower into the steaks and sprinkle with ground turmeric, dill, and sesame oil.
2. Put the steaks in the air fryer and cook at 365F for 7 minutes per side.

Per Serving: calories 75, fat 3.6, fiber 4.4, carbs 9.5, protein 3.5

10.Garlic Zucchini Slices

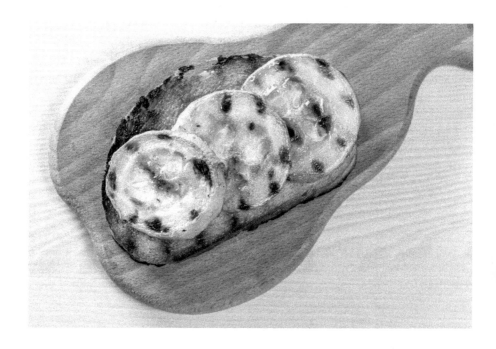

Prep Time:9 m | **Cook Time:** 6 m | **Servings:** 4

- 3 large zucchinis, sliced
- 1 tablespoon minced garlic
- 2 tablespoons sesame oil

1. Mix the sesame oil with minced garlic.
2. Then brush the zucchini slices with garlic mixture and put it in the air fryer.
3. Cook them for 3 minutes per side at 400F.

Per Serving: calories 166, fat 7.6, fiber 14.6, carbs 24.9, protein 4.2

11.Kale Saute

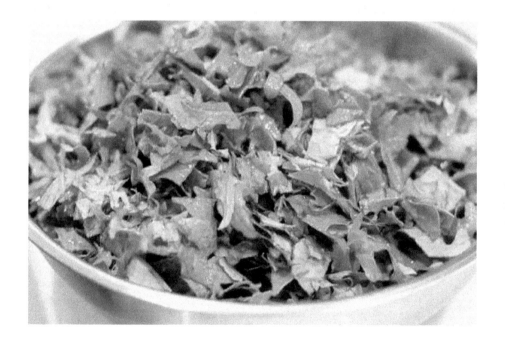

Prep Time:5 m | **Cook Time:** 10 m | **Servings:** 4

- 3 cups kale, torn
- 1 cup beef broth
- 1 oz almond, chopped
- ¼ cup mozzarella, shredded
- 1 teaspoon ghee
- 1 teaspoon dried oregano

1. Put all ingredients in the air fryer and gently mix with the help of the spoon.
2. Cook the saute at 360F for 10 minutes.

Per Serving: calories 91, fat 5.3, fiber 1.8, carbs 7.3, protein 4.8

12.Coriander Green Beans

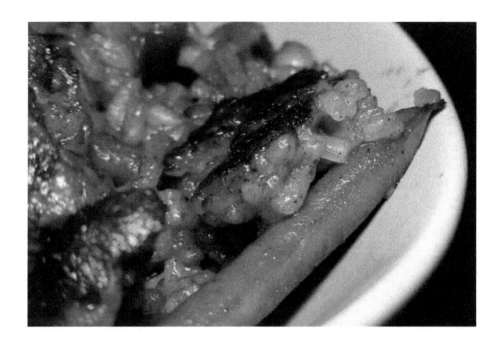

Prep Time:9 m | **Cook Time:** 6 m | **Servings:** 2

- 12 oz green beans, roughly chopped
- 1 tablespoon ground coriander
- 1 teaspoon salt
- 1 tablespoon coconut oil, melted

1. Mix green beans with ground coriander, salt, and coconut oil.
2. Put them in the air fryer and cook for 3 minutes per side and 400F.

Per Serving: calories 111, fat 7, fiber 5.8, carbs 12.2, protein 3.1

13.Crunchy Kale Leaves

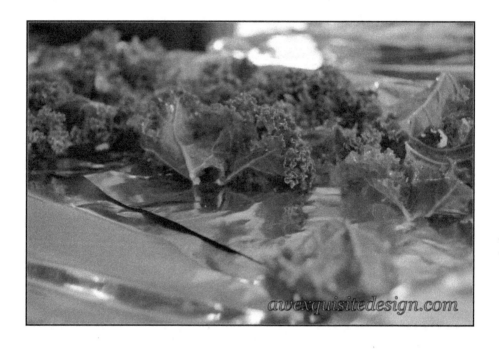

Prep Time:10 m | **Cook Time:** 12 m | **Servings:** 6

- 1 egg, beaten
- 1 teaspoon Per Serving yeast
- 1 teaspoon sesame oil
- 3 cups kale leaves, roughly chopped

1. Sprinkle the kale leaves with sesame oil, Per Serving yeast, and egg.
2. Carefully shake the leaves and put them in the air fryer.
3. Cook them at 400F for 12 minutes. Shake the leaves every 2 minutes to avoid burning.

Per Serving: calories 36, fat 1.5, fiber 0.6, carbs 3.8, protein 2.2

14.Vegetable Skewers

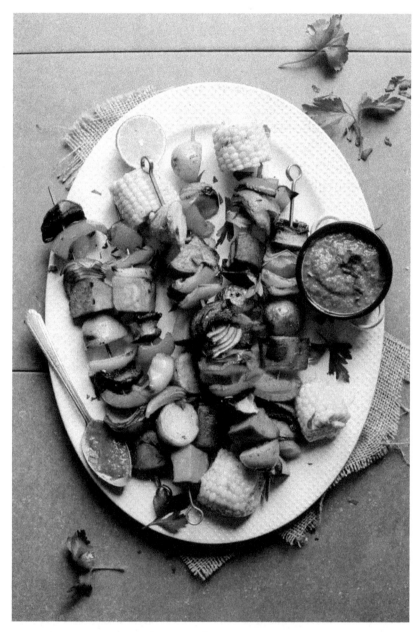

Prep Time:14 m | **Cook Time:** 14 m | **Servings:** 4

- 10 oz halloumi cheese, roughly chopped
- 1 zucchini, roughly chopped
- 1 jalapeno, roughly chopped
- 1 tomato, cut into 4 pieces
- 1 tablespoon olive oil
- ½ teaspoon dried rosemary

1. Sting the cheese, Zucchini, jalapeno, and tomato into the skewers and sprinkle with olive oil and dried rosemary.
2. Then, put the vegetable skewers in the air fryer and cook them at 375F for 14 minutes.

Per Serving: calories 300, fat 24.8, fiber 0.9, carbs 4.4, protein 16.1

15.Creamy Spinach

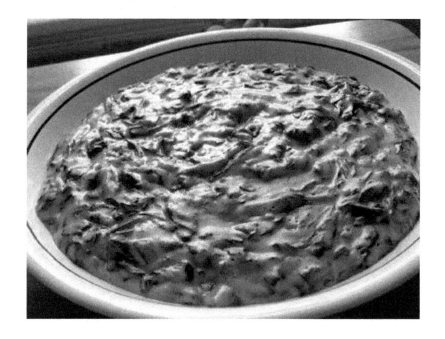

Prep Time:5 m | **Cook Time:** 15 m | **Servings:** 4

- 3 cups fresh spinach, chopped
- 1 cup heavy cream
- 1 oz macadamia nuts, chopped
- 1 tablespoon butter
- 1 teaspoon salt

1.Mix spinach with heavy cream, nuts, butter, and salt.
2. Put the spinach mixture in the ramekin and place the ramekin in the air fryer.
3. Cook the spinach at 350F for 15 minutes.

Per Serving: calories 185, fat 19.4, fiber 1.1, carbs 2.6, protein 1.9

16.Taco Broccoli Florets

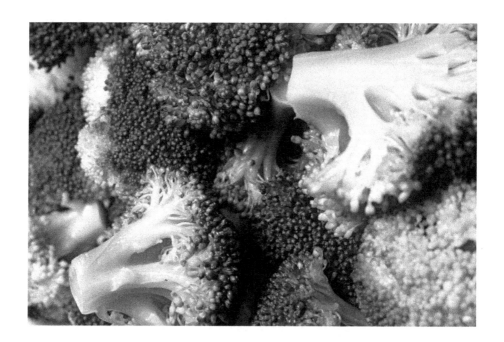

Prep Time:10 m | **Cook Time:** 12 m | **Servings:** 4

- 1-pound broccoli florets
- 1 tablespoon taco seasonings
- 2 tablespoons olive oil

1. Mix broccoli florets with taco seasonings and olive oil.
2. Put the broccoli in the air fryer and cook them at 375F for 12 minutes. Shake the vegetables after 6 minutes of cooking.

Per Serving: calories 106, fat 7.4, fiber 3, carbs 9, protein 3.2

17.Roasted Olives

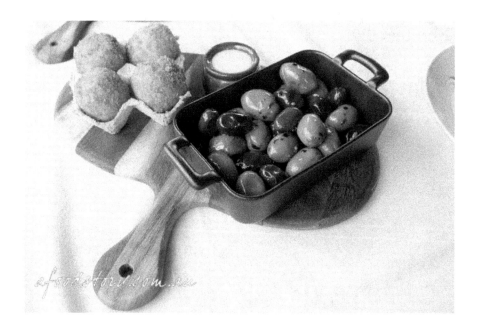

Prep Time:4 m | **Cook Time:** 2 m | **Servings:** 4

- 8 oz olives, pitted
- 1 teaspoon olive oil

1. Sprinkle olives with olive oil and put in the air fryer.
2. Cook them for 2 minutes per side at 400F.

Per Serving: calories 75, fat 7.2, fiber 1.8, carbs 3.6, protein 0.5

18.Roasted Mushroom Caps

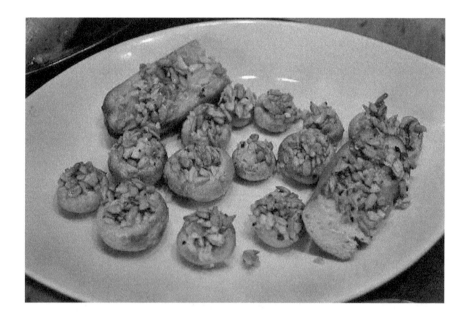

Prep Time:5 m | **Cook Time:** 15 m | **Servings:** 4

- 2-pounds mushroom caps
- 1 tablespoon avocado oil
- 1 teaspoon ground coriander

1. Put the mushrooms caps in the air fryer in one layer and sprinkle with avocado oil and ground coriander.
2. Cook the meal at 360F for 15 minutes.

Per Serving: calories 53, fat 1.1, fiber 2.7, carbs 7.7, protein 7.2

19.Cinnamon Garlic Cloves

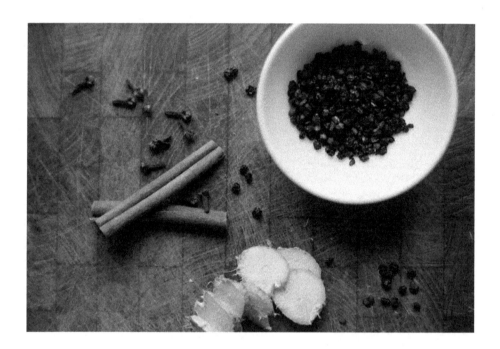

Prep Time:5 m | **Cook Time:** 10 m | **Servings:** 4

- 8 garlic cloves, peeled
- 2 tablespoons olive oil
- ¼ teaspoon dried thyme

1. Sprinkle the garlic cloves with olive oil and dried thyme, and put in the air fryer.
2. Cook the garlic at 350F for 10 minutes.

Per Serving: calories 69, fat 7, fiber 0.2, carbs 2, protein 0.4

20.Sautéed Celery Stalks

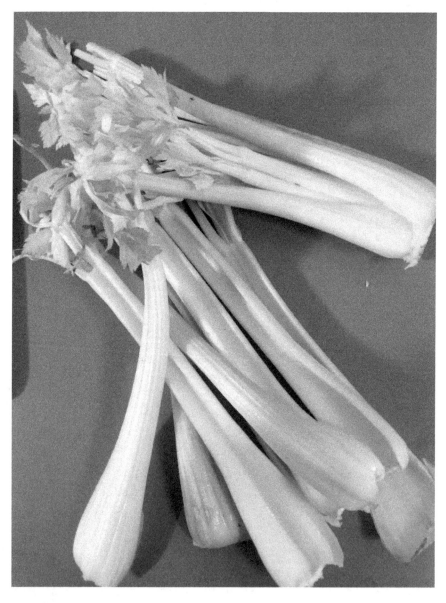

Prep Time:5 m | **Cook Time:** 10 m | **Servings:** 4

- 1-pound celery stalks, chopped
- ½ cup coconut cream
- 1 oz Parmesan, grated
- 1 teaspoon white pepper

1. Mix celery stalks with white pepper, parmesan, and coconut cream.
2. Put the vegetables in the air fryer and cook at 350F for 10 minutes.

Per Serving: calories 111, fat 8.9, fiber 2.6, carbs 5.6, protein 3.8

21.Keto Buffalo Cauliflower

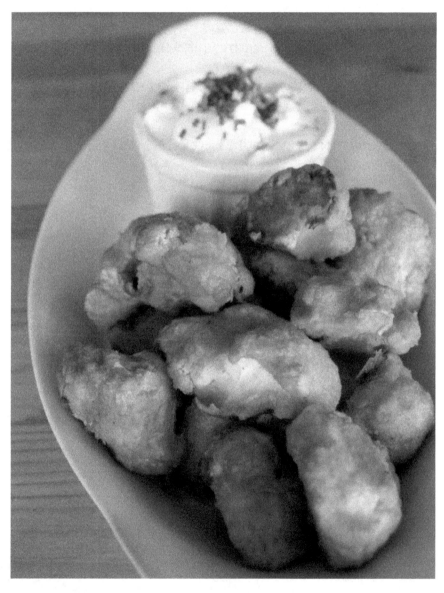

Prep Time:9 m | **Cook Time:** 6 m | **Servings:** 4

- 2 cups cauliflower florets
- ¼ cup coconut cream
- 2 tablespoons keto buffalo sauce
- 1 teaspoon olive oil

1. Mix cauliflower florets with coconut cream, buffalo sauce, and olive oil.
2. Put them in the air fryer and cook at 400F for 3 minutes per side.

Per Serving: calories 60, fat 4.8, fiber 1.8, carbs 4, protein 1.3

22.Bacon Brussels Sprouts

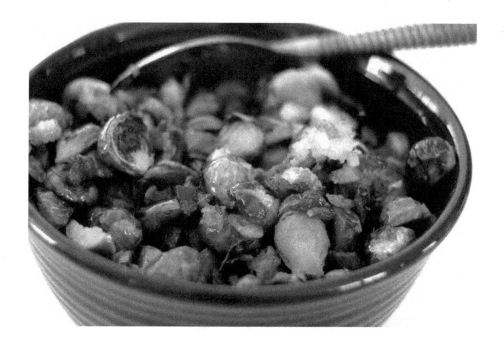

Prep Time:10 m | **Cook Time:** 15 m | **Servings:** 8

- 1 pound Brussels sprouts, trimmed
- 3 oz bacon, chopped
- 1 tablespoon coconut oil, melted
- 1 teaspoon salt

1. Mix Brussel sprouts with coconut oil and salt and put them in the air fryer.
2. Top the vegetables with bacon and cook at 360F for 15 minutes. Stir the vegetables from time to time to avoid burning.

Per Serving: calories 97, fat 6.3, fiber 2.1, carbs 5.3, protein 5.9

23.Coated Okra

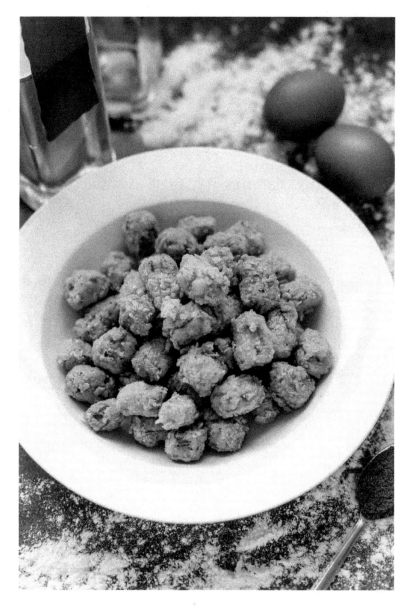

Prep Time: 14 m | **Cook Time:** 8 m | **Servings:** 4

- 1-pound okra, trimmed
- ½ cup coconut flour
- 3 eggs, beaten
- 1 teaspoon chili powder

1. Mix coconut flour with chili powder.
2. Then dip the okra in the eggs and coat it in the coconut flour mixture.
3. Put the okra in the air fryer and cook at 385F for 4 minutes per side.

Per Serving: calories 155, fat 5.1, fiber 9.9, carbs 19.1, protein 8.4

24.Roasted Artichoke Hearts

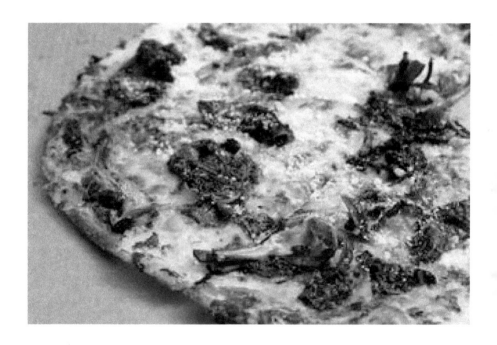

Prep Time:5 m | **Cook Time:** 15 m | **Servings:** 4

- 4 artichoke hearts, canned
- 1 teaspoon olive oil
- 1 tablespoon lemon juice
- 1 teaspoon ground black pepper

1. Sprinkle the artichoke hearts with olive oil, lemon juice, and ground black pepper.
2. Put them in the air fryer and cook for 15 minutes at 350F.

Per Serving: calories 88, fat 1.5, fiber 8.9, carbs 17.5, protein 5.4

25.Cajun Eggplants

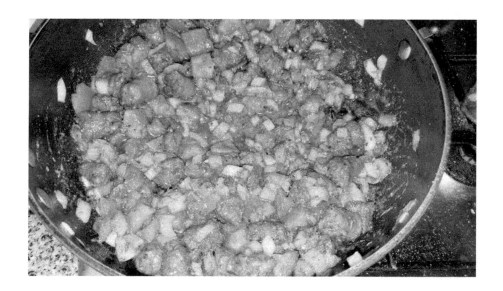

Prep Time:10 m | **Cook Time:** 15 m | **Servings:** 2

- 2 eggplants, roughly chopped
- 1 teaspoon Cajun seasonings
- 1 tablespoon sesame oil

1.Sprinkle the eggplants with Cajun seasonings and sesame oil.
2.Put the vegetables in the air fryer.
3.Cook them at 360F for 15 minutes.

Per Serving: calories 197, fat 7.8, fiber 19.3, carbs 32.2, protein 5.4

26.Topped Zucchini

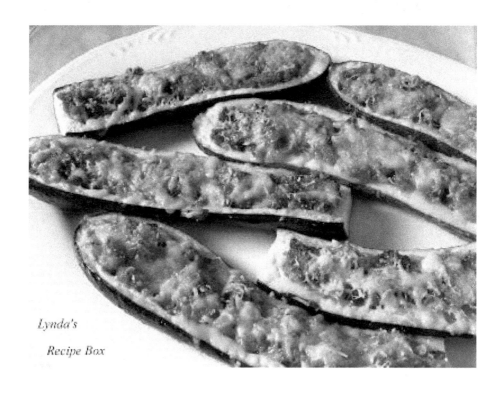

Lynda's

Recipe Box

Prep Time:5 m | **Cook Time:** 12 m | **Servings:** 2

- 1 large zucchini, trimmed, halved
- 1 teaspoon ground black pepper
- 1 cup Cheddar cheese, shredded
- 1 tablespoon olive oil
- ½ teaspoon dried parsley

1. Brush the air fryer basket with olive oil.
2. Put the Zucchini inside and sprinkle with ground black pepper.
3. Then top the Zucchini with Cheddar cheese and dried parsley.
4. Cook the meal at 375F for 12 minutes.

Per Serving: calories 316, fat 26, fiber 2.1, carbs 6.8, protein 16.1

27.Egg Green Beans

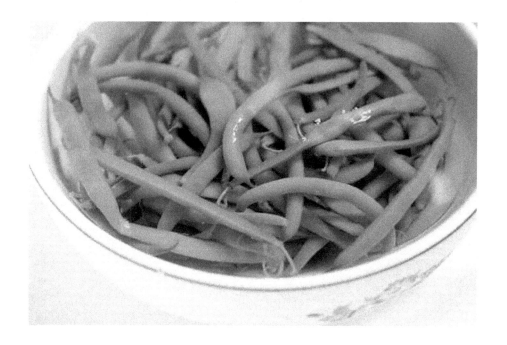

Prep Time: 15 m | **Cook Time:** 5 m | **Servings:** 2

- 10 oz green beans
- 2 eggs, beaten
- 2 tablespoons coconut shred
- 1 teaspoon ground turmeric
- Cooking spray

1. Sprinkle the green beans with eggs and turmeric.
2. Then sprinkle them with coconut shred and put in the air fryer.
3. Spray the green beans with cooking spray and cook at 400F for 5 minutes.

Per Serving: calories 161, fat 9.7, fiber 6.1, carbs 13.2, protein 8.2

28.Roasted Artichoke

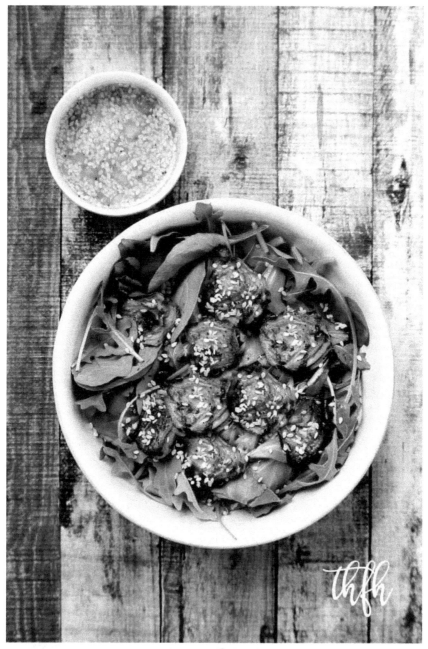

Prep Time:5 m | **Cook Time:** 15 m | **Servings:** 2

- 2 artichokes, trimmed
- 1 tablespoon olive oil
- 1 teaspoon onion powder

1. Put artichokes in the air fryer and sprinkle with onion powder and olive oil.
2. Cook the artichokes at 355F for 15 minutes.

Per Serving: calories 140, fat 7.3, fiber 8.8, carbs 18, protein 5.4

29.Cajun Okra

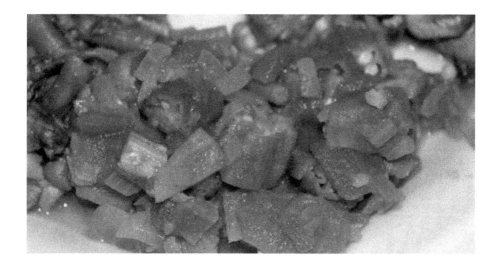

Prep Time:10 m | **Cook Time:** 10 m | **Servings:** 3

- 12 oz okra, chopped
- 1 teaspoon Cajun seasonings
- 1 tablespoon sesame oil

1. Mix okra with Cajun seasonings and sesame oil.
2. Put the vegetables in the air fryer and cook at 360F for 5 minutes.
3. Then shake the vegetables and cook them for 5 minutes more.

Per Serving: calories 85, fat 4.8, fiber 3.6, carbs 8.5, protein 2.2

30.Marinated Bell Peppers

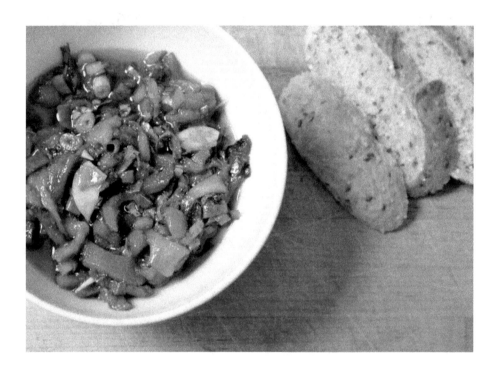

Prep Time:10 m | **Cook Time:** 5 m | **Servings:** 4

- 4 bell peppers, trimmed
- 1 tablespoon olive oil
- 1 teaspoon minced garlic
- 1 tablespoon apple cider vinegar

1. Sprinkle the bell peppers with olive oil and put them in the air fryer.
2. Cook the bell peppers at 400F for 5 minutes.
3. Then chop the bell peppers roughly and sprinkle with minced garlic and apple cider vinegar.

Per Serving: calories 70, fat 3.8, fiber 1.6, carbs 9.3, protein 1.2

31.Roasted Avocado Wedges

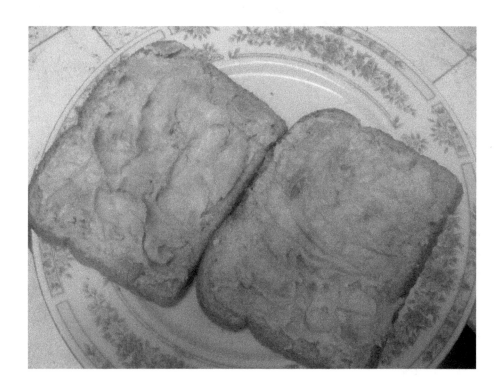

Prep Time:9 m | **Cook Time:** 6 m | **Servings:** 4

- 1 avocado, pitted, cut into 4 wedges
- 4 teaspoons coconut shred
- 1 egg, beaten
- ½ teaspoon ground nutmeg

1. Dip the avocado wedges in the egg and sprinkle with ground nutmeg.
2. Then sprinkle the avocado with coconut shred and put it in the air fryer.
3. Cook the meal at 400F for 3 minutes per side.

Per Serving: calories 136, fat 12.7, fiber 3.8, carbs 5.2, protein 2.4

32.Herbed Kalamata Olives

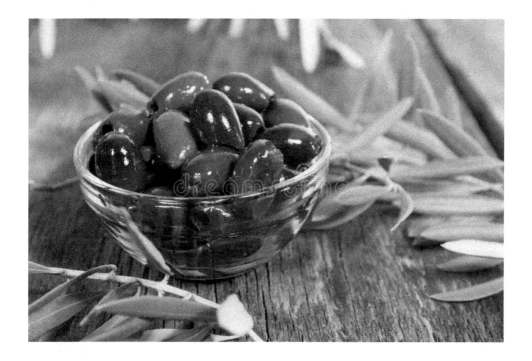

Prep Time:5 m | **Cook Time:** 7 m | **Servings:** 4

- 8 Kalamata Olives, pitted
- 1 teaspoon Italian seasonings
- 1 tablespoon olive oil
- 1 teaspoon coconut aminos

1. Sprinkle olives with Italian seasonings, olive oil, and coconut aminos.
2. Put the olives in the air fryer and cook at 360F for 8 minutes.

Per Serving: calories 45, fat 4.8, fiber 0.3, carbs 0.9, protein 0.1

33.Cauliflower Balls

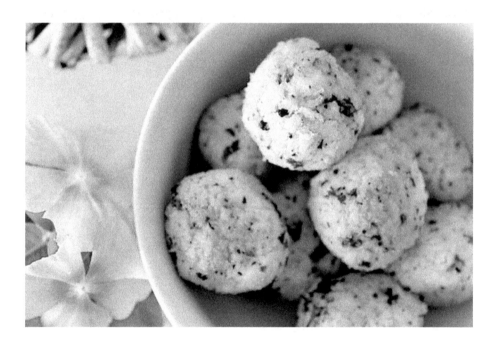

Prep Time: 15 m | **Cook Time:** 12 m | **Servings:** 4

- 2 cups cauliflower, shredded
- 3 tablespoons coconut flour
- 1 teaspoon ground cumin
- 2 tablespoons coconut oil
- 1 egg, beaten
- 1 teaspoon salt
- 1 teaspoon ground coriander
- 1 teaspoon dried basil
- Cooking spray

1. Mix shredded cauliflower with coconut flour, ground cumin, coconut oil, egg, salt, ground coriander, and dried basil.
2. Make the balls from the mixture and put them in the air fryer.
3. Spray the cauliflower balls with cooking spray and cook them at 385F for 6 minutes per side or until they are golden brown.

Per Serving: calories 134, fat 9.6, fiber 5.1, carbs 9, protein 4

34.Greek Style Olives

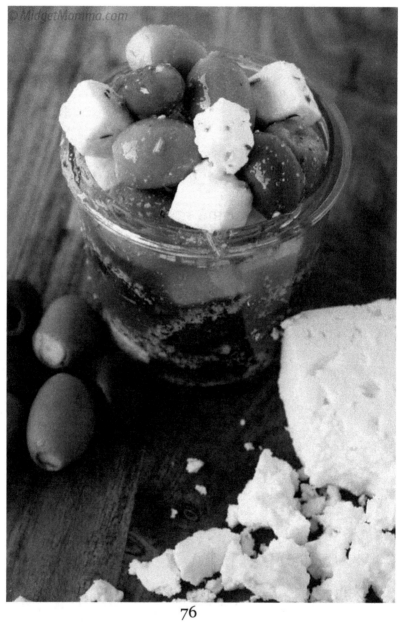

Prep Time:5 m | **Cook Time:** 12 m | **Servings:** 4

- 6 oz Feta cheese, crumbled
- 8 oz black olives, pitted
- 1 tablespoon coconut oil, melted
- 1 teaspoon dried thyme

1. Put olives in the air fryer and sprinkle with coconut oil and dried thyme.
2. Cook them at 350F for 12 minutes.
3. Sprinkle the cooked olives with crumbled Feta cheese.

Per Serving: calories 207, fat 18.5, fiber 1.9, carbs 5.5, protein 6.5

35.Zucchini Patties

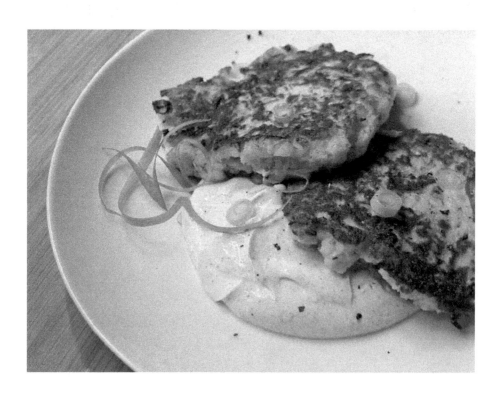

Prep Time: 14 m | **Cook Time:** 8 m | **Servings:** 4

- 2 zucchinis, grated
- 1 tablespoon dried dill
- 1 teaspoon cream cheese
- 1 cup almond flour
- 1 teaspoon salt
- Cooking spray

1. Mix zucchini with dried dill, cream cheese, almond flour, and salt
2. Make the patties from the zucchini mixture and put them in the air fryer.
3. Sprinkle the patties with cooking spray and cook at 375F for 4 minutes per side.

Per Serving: calories 189, fat 13.8, fiber 4.2, carbs 9.7, protein 7.4

36.Brussel Sprouts Roast

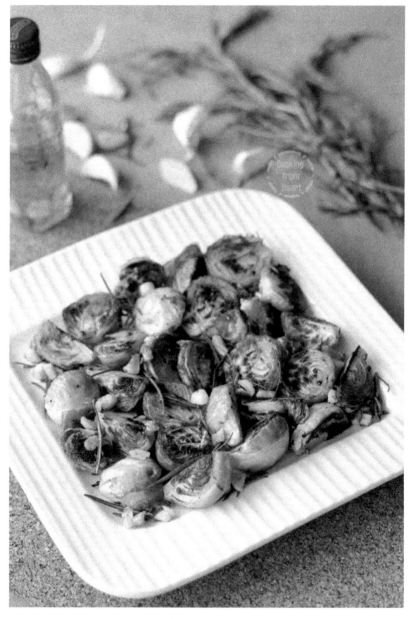

Prep Time:5 m | **Cook Time:** 12 m | **Servings:** 4

- 1-pound Brussel sprouts halved
- 1 tablespoon olive oil
- 1 teaspoon dried dill
- 2 oz Feta, crumbled

1. Mix Brussel sprouts with olive oil and dried dill.
2. Put the vegetables in the air fryer and cook at 375F for 6 minutes per side.
3. Top the cooked vegetables with crumbled feta.

Per Serving: calories 117, fat 6.9, fiber 4.3, carbs 11, protein 5.9

37.Broccoli Rice Balls

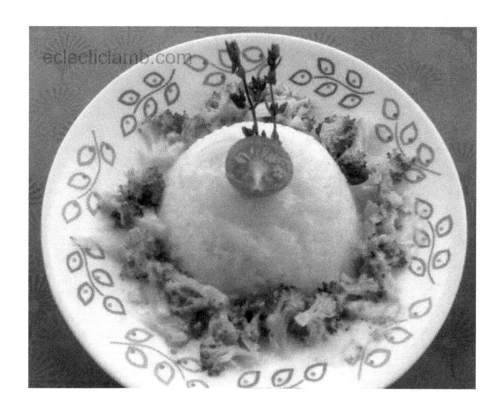

Prep Time:15 m | **Cook Time:** 5 m | **Servings:** 2

- 1 cup broccoli, shredded
- 3 oz Feta, crumbled
- 1 egg, beaten
- 1 tablespoon almond flour
- ½ teaspoon white pepper
- 1 teaspoon mascarpone
- 1 teaspoon avocado oil

1. Brush the air fryer basket with avocado oil.
2. Then mix all remaining ingredients and make the balls.
3. Put the balls in the air fryer in one layer and cook at 400F for 5 minutes.

Per Serving: calories 189, fat 13.7, fiber 1.8, carbs 6.2, protein 11.2

38.Cabbage Fritters

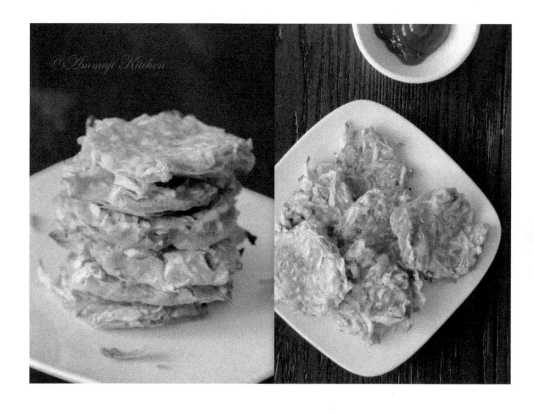

Prep Time:10 m | **Cook Time:** 12 m | **Servings:** 4

- 1 cup white cabbage, shredded
- 3 eggs, beaten
- 1 oz scallions, chopped
- 1/3 cup coconut flour
- 1 teaspoon cream cheese
- Cooking spray

1. Spray the air fryer basket with cooking spray from inside.
2. Then mix all remaining ingredients in the bowl.
3. Make the cakes from the cabbage mixture and put them in the air fryer basket in one layer.
4. Cook the cakes at 375F for 6 minutes per side.

Per Serving: calories 97, fat 4.6, fiber 4.6, carbs 8.5, protein 5.9

39.Broccoli Gnocchi

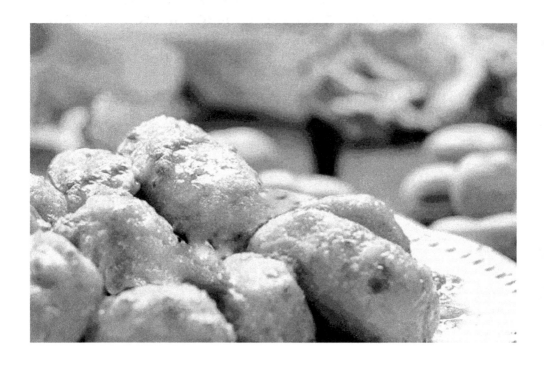

Prep Time:15 m | **Cook Time:** 4 m | **Servings:** 4

- 2 cups broccoli, chopped, boiled
- 2 oz provolone cheese, grated
- 1 egg, beaten
- 1 teaspoon white pepper
- 1 teaspoon mascarpone
- 3 tablespoons almond flour
- 1 tablespoon coconut oil
- 1 teaspoon dried parsley

1. Mix all ingredients in the mixing bowl until smooth.
2. Then, make the gnocchi and put them in the air fryer in one layer.
3. Cook the gnocchi at 400F for 2 minutes per side.

Per Serving: calories 146, fat 11.1, fiber 1.9, carbs 4.9, protein 7.6

40.Lemon Peppers

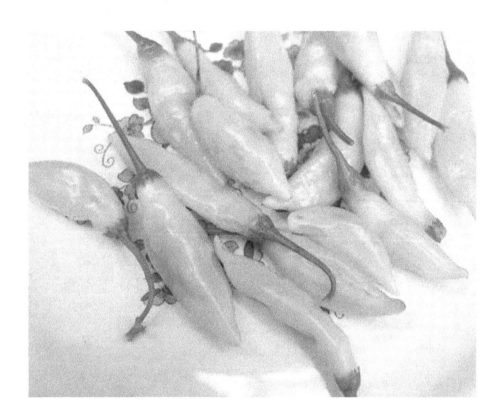

Prep Time: 5 m | **Cook Time:** 15 m | **Servings:** 4

- 2 cups bell peppers, roughly chopped
- 2 tablespoons lemon juice
- 1 teaspoon butter, softened
- 1 garlic clove, diced
- 1 teaspoon ground clove

1. Put the bell peppers in the air fryer basket and sprinkle with butter, garlic clove, and ground clove.
2. Cook the bell peppers for 15 minutes at 350F. Stir the peppers every 5 minutes to avoid burning.
3. Then transfer the cooked peppers to the bowl and sprinkle them with lemon juice.

Per Serving: calories 32, fat 1.3, fiber 1, carbs 5.2, protein 0.8

41.Portobello Steak

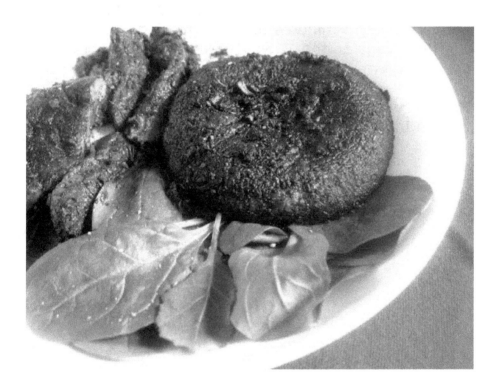

Prep Time:10 m | **Cook Time:** 5 m | **Servings:** 4

- 1-pound Portobello mushrooms
- 1 teaspoon ground coriander
- 4 teaspoons butter
- ½ teaspoon salt

1. Sprinkle the mushrooms with ground coriander, salt, and butter.
2. Put the mushrooms in the air fryer and cook for 5 minutes at 400F.

Per Serving: calories 61, fat 3.8, fiber 1.4, carbs 4.1, protein 4.1

42.Marinated roasted mushrooms

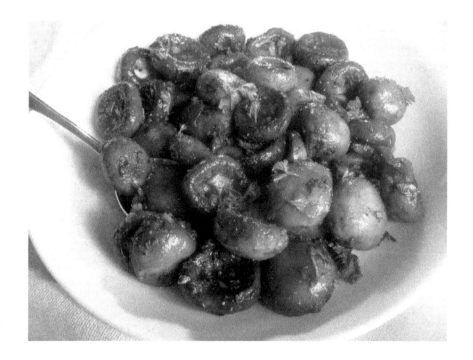

Prep Time10 m | **Cook Time** 13 m | **Serves:**6

- 10 ounces mushrooms
- 1 onion
- 1 garlic clove
- 1 ounce's bay leaf
- ¼ teaspoon black-eyed peas
- 3 tablespoons apple cider vinegar
- 1 tablespoon olive oil
- 1 teaspoon of sea salt
- 1 teaspoon ground black pepper

1. Peel the onion and garlic cloves. Slice the vegetables and sprinkle them with the black-eyed peas. Add the bay leaf and apple cider vinegar.
2. Chop the mushrooms and place them in the onion mixture. Add the sea salt and ground black pepper.
3. Mix well and let it rest for 10 minutes. Set the pressure cooker to Sauté mode. Pour the olive oil into the pressure cooker and add the mushroom mixture.
4. Close the pressure cooker lid and Sauté the dish for 13 minutes.
5. When the cooking time ends, open the pressure cooker lid and stir well.
6. Transfer the mushrooms to serving bowls.

Per Serving: Calories 189, Fats 3.2 g, Carbohydrates 42.64 g, Protein 5 g

43.Cauliflower puree with scallions

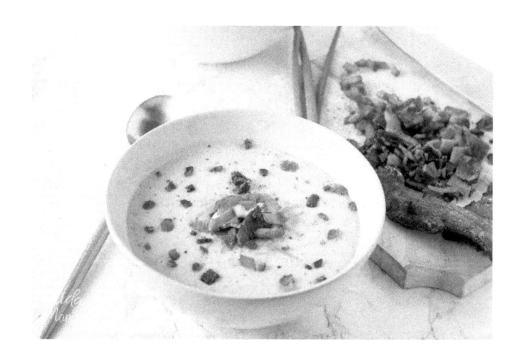

Prep Time 15 m | **Cook Time** 7 m | **Serves:** 6

- 1 head cauliflower
- 4 cups of water
- 1 tablespoon salt
- 4 tablespoons butter
- 3 ounces scallions
- 1 teaspoon chicken stock
- ¼ teaspoon sesame seeds
- 1 egg yolk

1. Wash the cauliflower and chop it roughly. Place the cauliflower in the pressure cooker.
2. Add the water and salt. Close the pressure cooker and cook the vegetables for 3 minutes.
3. Release the pressure and open the pressure cooker. Remove the cauliflower and let it rest briefly.
4. Place the cauliflower in a mixer. Add the butter the chicken stock, and the sesame seeds. Blend the mixture well.
5. Cut the scallions. Add the egg yolk to the mixer and blend the mixture for 25 seconds. Remove the puree from the blender and combine it with the scallions.

Per Serving: Calories 92, Fats 8.7 g, Carbohydrates 3.39 g, Protein 2 g

44.Vegetable tart

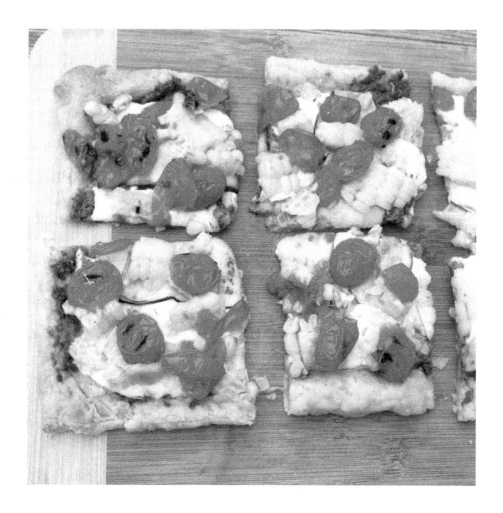

Prep Time 15 m | **Cook Time** 25 m | **Serves:** 9

- 7 ounces puff pastry
- 1 egg yolk
- 2 red bell peppers
- 5 ounces tomatoes
- 1 red onion
- 1 eggplant
- 3 ounces zucchini
- 1 teaspoon salt
- 1 teaspoon olive oil
- 1 teaspoon ground black pepper
- 1 tablespoon turmeric
- 7 ounces goat cheese
- ¼ cup cream

1. Whisk the egg yolk, combine it with the ground black pepper and stir well.
2. Roll the puff pastry using a rolling pin. Spray the pressure cooker with the olive oil inside and add the puff pastry.
3. Spread the puff pastry with the whisked egg. Chop the tomatoes and dice the onions. Chop the eggplants and Zucchini.
4. Combine the vegetables and sprinkle them with salt, turmeric, and cream. Mix well and place the vegetable mixture in the pressure cooker.
5. Chop the red bell peppers and sprinkle the pressure cooker mixture with them. Grate the goat cheese and sprinkle the tart with the cheese.
6. Close the pressure cooker lid Cook at Pressure mode for 25 minutes. When the dish is cooked, release the pressure and open the pressure cooker lid. Check if the tart is cooked and remove it from the pressure cooker.
7. Cut the tart into slices and serve it.

Per Serving: Calories 279, Fats 18.8 g, Carbohydrates 18.42 g, Protein 10 g

45.Zucchini pizza

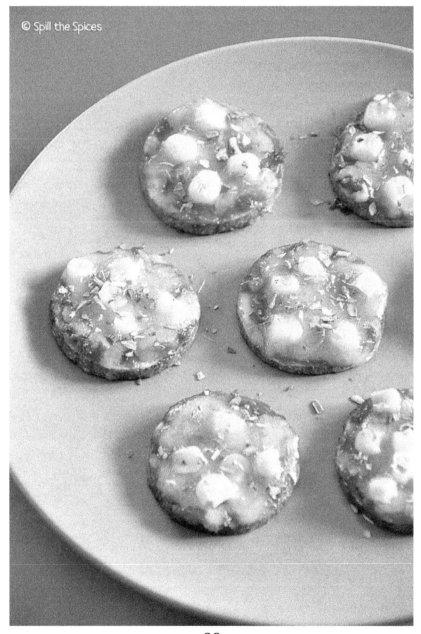

Prep Time 10 m | **Cook Time** 8 m | **Serves:** 2

- 1 zucchini
- ½ teaspoon tomato paste
- 5 oz Parmesan, shredded
- ½ teaspoon chili flakes
- ¼ teaspoon dried basil
- 1 teaspoon olive oil

1. Cut the Zucchini into halves to get boards. Then scoop the flesh from them and spread with the tomato paste from inside.
2. After this, fill Zucchini with the shredded cheese. Sprinkle them with chili flakes, dried basil, and olive oil.
3. Put the zucchini pizzas in the cooker and close the lid.
4. Cook the pizzas on-air crisp mode at 375F for 8 minutes.

Per Serving: Calories 331, Fats 21.9 g, Carbohydrates 6 g, Protein 28.1 g

46.Black beans in tomato sauce

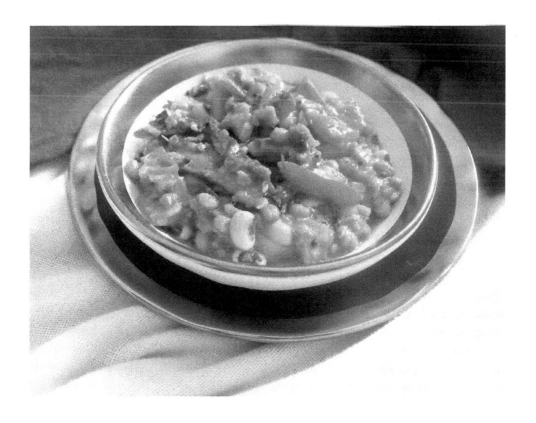

Prep Time 10 m | **Cook Time** 19 m | **Serves:** 7

- 8 ounces black beans
- 1 onion
- 1 cup tomato paste
- 1 tablespoon minced garlic
- 1 teaspoon ground black pepper
- 4 ounces celery stalk
- 4 cups chicken stock
- 1/2 teaspoons chile pepper
- ½ teaspoon turmeric

1. Place the black beans in the pressure cooker. Peel the onion and chop it. Add the tomato paste, garlic, ground black pepper.
2. Chicken stock chile pepper and turmeric in the pressure cooker. Mix well and close the pressure cooker lid.
3. Cook the dish on Pressure mode for 15 minutes. When the cooking time ends, release the pressure and open the pressure cooker lid.
4. Add the chopped onion and mix well. Cook the dish in Sauté mode for 4 minutes.
5. Open the pressure cooker lid and mix well. Transfer the cooked dish to a serving bowl.

Per Serving: Calories 109, Fats 2.1 g, Carbohydrates 17.59 g, Protein 6 g

47.Roasted veggie mix

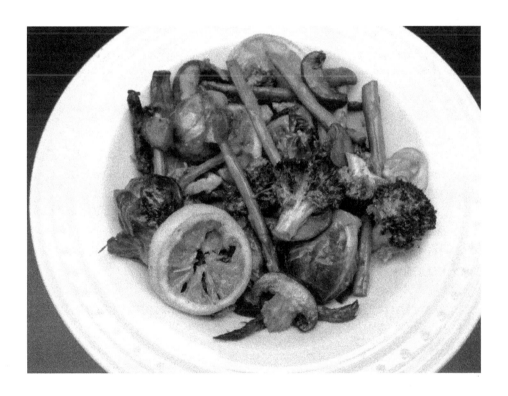

Prep Time 10 m | **Cook Time** 30 m | **Serves:** 10

- 2 eggplants
- 2 yellow bell peppers
- 1 tablespoon salt
- 8 ounces tomatoes
- 2 turnips
- 1 zucchini
- 1 tablespoon oregano
- 2 carrots
- 3 tablespoons sesame oil
- 4 cups beef broth

1. Peel the eggplants and chop them. Sprinkle the eggplants with salt and stir well. Remove the seeds from the bell peppers and chop them.
2. Slice the tomatoes and chop turnips. Chop the Zucchini.
3. Peel the carrots and grate them. Transfer all the vegetables to the pressure cooker. Add the oregano, sesame oil, and beef broth.
4. Mix well and close the pressure cooker lid. Cook the dish on Steam mode for 30 minutes.
5. When the cooking time ends, transfer the dish to serving bowls.

Per Serving: Calories 107, Fats 5 g, Carbohydrates 13.2 g, Protein 4 g

48.Summertime Veggie Soup

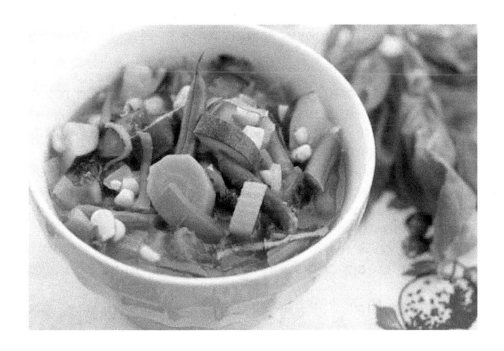

Prep Time 10 m | **Cook Time** 3 m | **Serves:** 6

- 3 cups leeks, sliced
- 6 cups rainbow chard, stems and leaves, chopped
- 1 cup celery, chopped
- 2 tablespoons garlic, minced
- 1 teaspoon dried oregano
- 1 teaspoon salt
- 2 teaspoons fresh ground black pepper
- 3 cups chicken broth
- 2 cups yellow summer squash, sliced into 1/ inch slices ¼ cup fresh parsley, chopped
- ¾ cup heavy whip cream 4-6 tablespoons parmesan cheese, grated

1.Add leeks, chard, celery, 1 tablespoon garlic, oregano, salt, pepper, and broth to your Air fryer
2.Lock lid and cook on high pressure for 3 minutes. Quick-release pressure
3.Open the lid and add more broth, set your pot to Saute mode, and adjust heat to high
4.Add yellow squash, parsley, and remaining 1 tablespoon garlic
5. Let it cook for 2-3 minutes until the squash is soft
5.Stir in cream and sprinkle parmesan. Serve and enjoy!

Per Serving: Calories: 210, Fat: 14g, Carbohydrates: 10g, Protein: 10g

49.Simple Rice Cauliflower

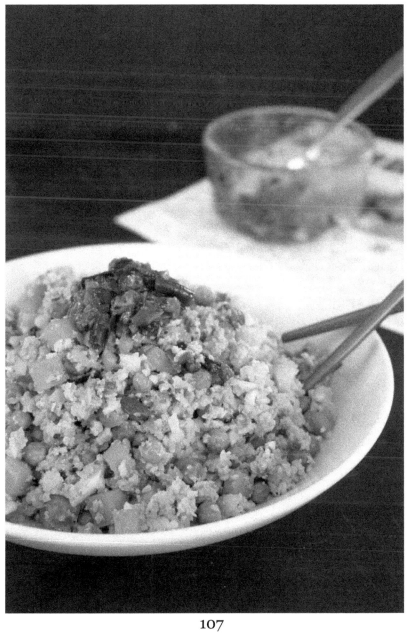

Prep Time 10 m | **Cook Time** 15 m | **Serves:** 4

- 1 large cauliflower head
- 2 tablespoons olive oil
- ¼ teaspoon salt
- ½ teaspoon dried parsley
- ½ teaspoon cumin
- ¼ teaspoon turmeric
- ¼ teaspoon paprika
- Fresh cilantro
- Lime wedges
- Directions

1.. Wash the cauliflower and trim the leaves
2.. Place a steamer rack on top of the pot and transfer the florets to the rack
3. Add 1 cup of water into the air fryer. Lock up the lid and cook on HIGH pressure for 1 minute
4. Once done, do a quick release. Transfer the flower to a serving platter
5. Set your pot to Saute mode and add oil; allow the oil to heat up
6. Cook the flowers
7. Season with a bit of salt. Squize a bit of lime

Per Serving: Calories: 160, Fat: 14g, Carbohydrates: 8g, Protein: 3g

50.Spicy Cauliflower Steak

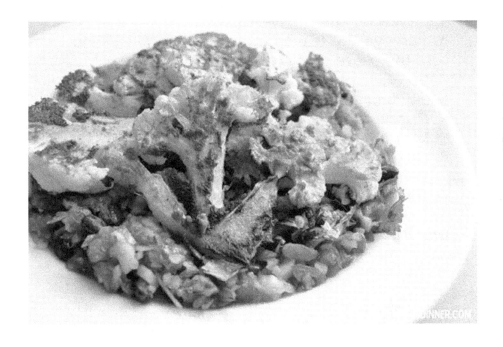

Prep Time 10 m | **Cook Time** 4 m | **Serves:** 6

- 1 large head cauliflower
- 2 tablespoon extra-virgin olive oil
- 2 teaspoons paprika
- 2 teaspoon ground cumin
- ¾ teaspoon kosher salt
- 1 cup fresh cilantro, chopped
- 1 lemon, quartered

1. Place the steamer rack into your Air fryer. Add 1 and a ½ cups of water
2. Remove the leaves from the cauliflower and trim the core to ensure that it can sit flat
3. Carefully place it on the steam rack. Take a small bowl and add olive oil, cumin, paprika, salt
4. Drizzle the mixture over the cauliflower
5. Lock up the lid and cook on high pressure for 4 minutes
6. Quick release the pressure. Slice into 1-inch steaks
7. Divide the mixture among serving plates and sprinkle with cilantro. Serve and enjoy!

Per Serving: Calories: 283, Fats: 19g, Carbohydrates: 18g, Protein: 10g

CPSIA information can be obtained
at www.ICGtesting.com
Printed in the USA
LVHW080235150321
681561LV00006B/152